HOW TO BECOME A REAL HOLISTIC HEALTH PRACTITIONER:

LEARN THE INSIDER'S SECRETS AND WHERE MOST EDUCATIONAL INSTITUTES FAIL

Copyright 2020, David D. Jameson, DNM

ISBN: 9798556999930

P.S. I am sure you will notice that I don't refer to my people as "patients." The word patient implies sickness. My people are not sick; they have simply stepped off their old path and onto a new one.

TABLE OF CONTENTS

ACKNOWLEDGMENTS

To my Family, my Friends, my Blue Lotus Family, my editorial staff, and

all holistic practitioners and supporters from the alpha to the omega.

My hope is for all to enjoy "the other side of health."

Come to the cliff, he said.

They said, we are afraid.

Come to the cliff, he said.

They came.

He pushed them.

And they flew.

INTRODUCTION

BECOMING A HOLISTIC HEALTH PRACTITIONER—A GLIMPSE BEHIND THE CURTAIN

"The Warrior-Sage admits to his ignorance and holds on to nothing. In doing so, he has access to everything."
Stuart Wilde, The Quickening

When I completed my doctorate of natural medicine, I thought I had all the answers—or at least enough of them to get people better.

However, when that diploma was handed to me, I could not have been more wrong. I would soon discover myself to be a fraud. Well, not really. I'd done all the course work and proven myself quite successful, by all traditional accounts. But I had only learned a fraction of what I needed to truly heal—or even help—anyone. And with that as my goal, how could I settle with only a cursory knowledge of a topic so crucial?

If I were ever to help anyone get to the root cause of illness, I'd soon learn I needed a lot more. I'd need to understand not only the parts of the body, what diseases existed, and what medications to prescribe, as I already had—but I'd need to know what *wellness* actually is, not just from reading a few articles, but from living and breathing it. And I'd need to know the secrets that Western medicine didn't so much as whisper to me in med school; yet by making the right observations—and with the right mentors—they were screaming at me all along.

Ask, and you shall receive. It seemed like the secrets to healing lay just beyond the curtain. And even when I had the medical degree to get behind the curtain, I knew there was more to it than what I could initially see.

So I became obsessed with the ancient teaching of Ayurveda and all the miracles that come from this way of life. People want a magical pill to vanquish every ailment. If you want to mask symptoms instead of pulling the problem up by the roots, then go ahead and pop that pill. But it's only a matter of time before the problem will come back tenfold. Ayurveda involves changing your daily habits, your routine, so that wellness becomes you, from the inside out. Is it as easy to do as popping a pill? No, it takes work. But is it simple to grasp? Absolutely, and fluency comes with practice.

That drive to pursue wellness—not just disease and pharmaceuticals—is why I pursued becoming a *holistic health practitioner* (which we refer to as HHP on our website when discussing our certification program), on top of my existing medical degree.

And it is why, once I found the right holistic health institute, I couldn't stop there. I needed to share what I knew—rather than just keep it all to myself. If you held the answers to so many of life's problems, wouldn't you be compelled to share them with everyone, too? If you are reading this book, I'm guessing you are like me: you want to be part of the solution.

I was so in love with this healing philosophy that I bought the institute I attended—once known as OM Wellness Institute, now known as Blue Lotus Institute for Holistic Studies—and now I run it, to teach others like you. We offer a Certified Holistic

Health Professional program that is second to none—and the only prerequisite is that you need to care enough about the well-being of yourself and others that you choose to enroll. You will walk away with a diploma—and a new lens to see things you never saw before.

We vow to perpetually improve our programs as new findings come out, while keeping its age-old wisdom. I vow to share with my students ALL I can to help.

You may be a physician or provider yourself. Or you may be someone who, like me, knows there is more to health than what you read in a textbook or pharmaceutical pamphlet.

At Blue Lotus Institute for Holistic Studies, we welcome anyone with a passion for learning about *true health and healing.* We welcome doctors, healthcare workers (like nurses, chiropractors, naturopaths, dieticians, practice administrators, and more), nutrition/vitamin store owners, massage therapists, fitness and yoga instructors, medical/healthcare salespeople, and "average Joes and Janes" who are passionate about improving lives—for themselves and those around them. Even if you've already worked as a holistic health practitioner, you will learn more through our program than in any other.

And if you've never held a medical degree or even a degree at all, that's okay too. We address mind, body, and spirit—teaching best practices from all walks of life—so you can practice the rare art and science of true holistic health. I'm not afraid to be a little edgy in pursuing fields others might not touch, because I'm that passionate about getting it right. But I will also teach you the age-old practices that other programs neglect, so you have a foundation that predates anything I could have discovered on my own.

This book introduces the true practice of being a holistic health practitioner. But it goes beyond, to explore the niche areas I found to be obliterated in any classrooms I'd seen before entering this Institute. Learn from my mistakes, and repeat my successes, to shortcut your path to freedom and health.

Should you choose to explore our Holistic Health Practitioner Certification at Blue Lotus Institute for Holistic Studies after reading this book, you should know we've made enrolling and participating as simple as possible. Since it is online-based, the program accommodates those who work full-time. It will show you how not only to *study* the healing arts, but to *practice* them. The program allows for an easy transition once you are done, as you move from student to holistic health practitioner. Or if you are already a holistic health practitioner, you will reap the benefits as you go, with practical information to apply immediately.

I believe in our Institute so strongly that I'm offering you a FREE gift at the end of this book, valued at $250. You can skip to the end now if you want, but I hope the promise of that offer won't stop you from gleaning all you can from this book in the meantime.

In fact, please ask yourself:

- *Do you truly want to provide healing and well-being to others—and take your own health to a new level?*

- *Or do you want to stay in the complacency that you know isn't enough—only to find yourself here again next year, one year older and further into a career or life that isn't fulfilling you or your clients/patients/customers/family?*

If you are ready for a change *now*, get ready to dive in, because here we go. The journey of thousands of years begins in the pages of this simple book. Shall we begin?

David D. Jameson, DNM

Doctor of Natural Medicine
Certified Ayurvedic Practitioner
Certified Holistic Health Practitioner
Clinic: www.bluelotushealingcenter.com
810.620.1000
Blue Lotus Institute for Holistic Studies
www.holistichealthpractitioner.com
800.385.8371

CHAPTER 1

SHOULD YOU?

"It's a paradox that to be healthy, you must be healthy."

David D. Jameson, DNM

Doctor of Natural Medicine

If you've read to this point, you are probably curious enough to ask yourself: "Should I become a holistic health practitioner—or further my practice with more education?" or maybe just, "What is this Dr. Dave on about?"

When I started practicing holistic health, I made the rookie error of believing I'd arrived at my final destination. However, it didn't take me long to realize I'd only scratched the surface.

Becoming a holistic health practitioner involves more than taking a few classes and walking away with a framed sheet of paper with your name on it. If you're interested in that sort of quick recognition, I recommend that you take a Dale Carnegie or John Maxwell workshop.

Those options are cheaper and far easier than mastering holistic health and all its benefits.

Holistic health requires an inside-out approach to healing, reaffirming the ancient texts that tell us we must *work on ourselves first*. Until you are ready to dig deep inside yourself first, you will remain unable to help anyone else.

Unwilling to do anything half-heartedly, once I started, I dove eagerly down the rabbit hole of holistic health. I found a magical place where health and happiness not only intersected—but seemed interchangeable.

When you see someone enjoying true happiness, you also see a strong element of natural health. Likewise, when you see someone enjoying their natural health, isn't that person typically happy?

If an average person found a genie granting two wishes, most would ask for *wealth*—as well as *happiness* or *health*.

Do you know why people automatically ask for wealth? Because most people believe *if they possess enough wealth, they can buy health and happiness.*

Go to any bookstore, and you'll see shelves of books with the words *happiness* or *health* in the titles. Who does not want more happiness and health? Sadly, pursuing happiness and health can look a lot like chasing steam: the more you try to grab it, the more it evades your grasp. Isn't happiness as we think of it nothing more than the absence of misery, as the great scholars Osho, Buddha, and Epicurus suggest?

Remember that I said that holistic health requires an inside-out approach. To find happiness and health, we must first practice an outside-in approach.

"I'm bored," a person might say when confronting boredom, which is misery in a passive state. "I know! I'll watch TV!" Don't we all try to alter our *internal* unhappiness by manipulating our *external* environment?

"It feels like I have some inflammation going on," a person might say. "I know! I'll take some turmeric!" And just like that, we try to change our *internal* state by taking something from the outside.

I am not critical of people who buy into the outside-in path to happiness and health. Instead, I feel sorry for them. Hell, from the moment we're born, we learn that the best way to feel better on the inside is to manipulate our external environment. A baby cries until someone in the external environment offers a nipple, bottle, diaper change, or hug. A toddler acts up until the external environment snaps to attention and gives him a toy or plops him down in front of the television. Since birth, our programming leads us to believe there's an easy external fix for whatever ails us.

I knew I wanted to pursue the holistic health practitioner path when I began realizing that happiness and health are synonymous states that come from within. I didn't want to become the master of manipulating the external environment; rather, I wanted to master my internal environment first. Then, and only then, could I teach others to do the same, transformative, inside-out work for themselves.

Be "Perfect," Be Aware

Imagine jumping into a mountain-fed river in early spring. That'll wake you up in a hurry, especially if you anticipated the water would feel like a plunge into the shallows of a sun-drenched ocean in summer. That river leap instead sends biting pain into your body—as the icy, winter runoff chills your bones, taking your breath away.

Do you know what else creates pain? Realizing that up to this point, you've been bullshitting yourself.

The bullshit I'm talking about is when you try to convince yourself and others that you're healthy and happy when you're not. The HOLISTIC HEALTH PRACTITIONER can't just appear healthy or look like someone who is happy. You have to *be perfect*, and that starts with being *aware.*

Did you cringe when I said that you must be *perfect*? If you did, that's okay. We all know that perfection is impossible. But you must embody *the desire to be perfect*, because your patients and clients will know if you don't. And they deserve—and need—a practitioner who is striving for the impossible. Lead by example, even if that threshold seems beyond reach.

When you think of Buddha, Jesus, Osho, Hippocrates, and other scholars, you imagine they had it all figured out. You imagine they were perfect in every way, that they embody the unattainable. And yet, we try to live like these great leaders before us. As a practitioner, you also need to put yourself in a position that feels unreachable, to truly help those in need. You need to give them a goal to push their own limits beyond belief.

Imagine the potential, if you inspired your patients and community from a place of desiring—and even expecting—such perfection to form in the lives of those you serve. What if you could spark the right change, just by striving for something better? What if seeing your example leads someone to become aware of what needs changing?

About 80 percent of all changes we make in our lives start with that "A-ha!" of awareness.

Do you know what makes awareness so difficult? Our training tells us to practice understanding, even enabling to a point, where we give ourselves and others an out. So instead of helping others develop their own self-awareness, we give them excuses like, "Oh, well that's just Jimmy. He's got a real sweet tooth!" Or "Poor Jenny. She loves her snacks!" Or "Dale does have his days and nights mixed up. He's just a night owl."

We give these behaviors titles and labels (which is another way of saying *outs* and *excuses*), and we tell our clients that it's OK. And let me tell you one reason we do that using myself as an example. When I first started down the path of becoming a holistic health practitioner, it didn't take me long to realize that I did all of those same things myself around my own behavior. If health and happiness are synonymous, and I believe they are, it's simple to understand why we let so many patently unhealthy behaviors into our lives—and into the lives of our clients. We permit behaviors that give us *temporary reprieve from our momentary misery.*

Ancient philosophers would argue that true happiness is actually unstable, because it means we must use one moment to refine the next. And those moments can change our state. Instead of happiness, I learned about bliss. Unlike happiness, which is merely the absence of misery, bliss is a continual state that does not change with external stressors. No matter what comes in, we can keep our emotional state fixed on bliss. Have you ever noticed that in most photographs of the Dalai Lama, he's giggling? Life is like a big joke to him. He's in a perpetual state of bliss, where his emotions remain detached from a yo-yo of mood swings.

If you're on social media, take thirty minutes some day and look at every single post out there. Unless you've curated a following of like-minded people only, you will find opinions shared on any platform you strongly oppose. But did you know it's possible to read those contrary opinions, even those that seemed laced with venom, and not respond? Did you know you can also read opinions you disagree with while your breathing and heart rate remain unchanged? Bliss is not dependent upon any external element. And the best news is that you don't have to be the Dalai Lama to achieve the state of bliss.

So where do you start on the journey to becoming a holistic health practitioner? *Look in the mirror, and identify where you've been going wrong.*

In my case, I realized that my athletic training prepared me to be tough and work hard without any show of emotion. To be clearer, I played rugby. Do you get the picture? Yeah, I hit guys with all I had, with no consequence. I even got so into the game that I refereed. But I also played baseball—a precision sport. Rugby taught me to be tough, while baseball tuned my focus and leadership skills. And both sports taught me how to work as a team.

But the problem with any sport is it's based on competition, which easily leads to an aggressive mindset—requiring that you offset it with something to find balance. For me, that something was drinking. As a "kid," I foolishly thought I could drown my problems—and my tension. But drinking only led to serious mental imbalances. I wasn't managing my internal pressure in a way that was sustainable or healthy. I was only masking symptoms—as I ran from my own inner peace.

Once I embraced a more peaceful mindset, I could embody the right type of stoicism—not masking the tension, but managing it. The pressure was released, and my body started to change. I had always been prone to rashes. But once I calmed my mind, my rashes got better.

Native Americans understood the mind-body connection. Medicine men were put through a string of very difficult challenges during the first half of their lives. If they were able to come through and understand these obstacles, they developed the power to change the second half of their lives. The medicine man, the healer, could intuitively sense the wellness of others, relate to them, and help them. Real holistic health practitioners serve as modern day medicine men and women, because they own the full spectrum of wellness.

You'll note that the subtitle of this book is, *Where Most Educational Institutes Fail*. Here's why I believe they fail: they never go past the academic surface of wellness. Traditional doctors take courses and pass tests with little or no human interaction. As a result, doctors receive certificates to hang on their walls to "prove" they've learned something of value.

Let me tell you, *those credentials mean next to nothing.*

My approach involves *seeing and hearing the whole person*. I would much rather look at my students to see how they write, or listen to them list the medications they're taking and all the specialists they are seeing, as this gives me insight into how they are doing as a whole. As Hippocrates said, "It's more important to know what sort of person has a disease than to know what sort of disease a person has." People with cancer tend to live longer when they don't know they have cancer, you know? This scenario happened to my friend. When he learned he had cancer, he gave up and gave into death. And that's exactly what came for him. I'm not suggesting we mask cancer, but we do need to tap into the power that keeps people well. So I want to know everything about a person I am helping. I want to know that they are doing something to help themselves. I want to know the things they don't even yet know about themselves, but which I can see—and ultimately shape—if I observe them. Because if they can't know and help themselves, how can they help anyone else?

Changing Physiologically

Just like Gandhi said, "Be the change you wish to see in the world." If you want to be a true holistic health practitioner, you must *be that change*, because that change snowballs to improve the quality of lives for those we serve.

My desire to *be the change* led me to own and operate my own center— Blue Lotus Institute for Holistic Studies.

As a final note, don't confuse a real holistic health practitioner with a holistic health theorist. Theory is cheap, to modify a well-known phrase. But *doing* is a completely different animal.

For me, to sign a diploma or certificate after attending our program, you have to prove that you've gone from a health practitioner into a true *holistic* health practitioner. You must show that you've experienced well-being from the inside-out. You must prove to me that your commitment is solid, and that this is your new way of life.

We will explore the four modules of the program throughout this book—giving you a taste of what you will learn. But first, I want to make sure you understand the foundation of what you need to make this work.

Whenever you board an airplane, the flight attendant gives you a speech about putting on your mask. Do you remember what the flight attendant says? "Put on your own mask first; then, help those around you." If you want my name certifying that you truly "get it," I need to know that you get it well enough that you can and will help others put on their own masks, so to speak.

No, I won't promise to make the process easy. The path to becoming a real holistic health practitioner should require hard work, so you know that you've accomplished something meaningful and of value. All the other courses that I've ever seen are strictly institutional. You take a class, and voila, you get a certificate to put on your wall. But besides that certificate, you have little else of value to offer. You still need your hand held to actually initiate any change.

When I graduated from the Institute, I knew it was unique. I actually went to owning my own business shortly after receiving my certificate. Who can say that? It had such an impact on me, that I bought the institute, and now I run it.

The difference? Blue Lotus Institute for Holistic Studies teaches practitioners *to live health before practicing*. Our students see what works and doesn't. They apply their learnings with their (willing) family and friends. Maybe they will learn what it's like not to eat so close to bedtime, and see how that affects their sluggishness in the morning. Or maybe they will wake up at 6:00 a.m. to practice breath work and yoga, and see how much focus and energy they have the rest of the day. We ask students to take health into their own hands—instead of sweeping that topic under the rug, as is done in nearly every other program I've encountered. We don't want you to be like the dentist with bad teeth. We want you to embody the program—so you can reap its rewards and model them for others. We want to equip you to handle most health crises without ever setting foot in an M.D.'s office.

Do you know what most wanna-be practitioners find is the hardest part? Taking that first, honest look in the mirror. Then, and only then, will you be equipped to turn your life around to a new paradigm and way of living.

I've found no other way to live, and I know of no other way to help others, than to focus inward first—and then expand that knowledge and awareness to those we serve.

Getting back to the title of this chapter: *Who should become a holistic health practitioner?* We discussed in the introduction some of the typical paths that people come from—other medical practices/positions, owners of businesses in wellness/healthcare, and family members of those who are suffering. To put it more simply, I believe firmly that this is the right path for you if—

- You want to take a deep look inside yourself
- You wish to be the change in the world, one that leads others to improved well-being
- You desire to be of benefit and service to others.

If this stirs something in your soul, I believe you've already begun your journey. And unlike other programs, given our Institute's flexible online modules, you don't need to quit your job or even make this your new vocation. I've certified engineers and grocery store clerks, doctors and midwives. You're on the right path if you want to learn more about yourself, improve the health of your family, and change lives.

How did I know I needed to make this program part of my destiny? When I saw that this Institute came up for sale, I jumped all in, screaming aloud, "Yes! This is what I've been looking for!" And it changed my life.

Should you dive in and learn from this program, too? If you've read this far, the answer is likely yes. If you want to help yourself and others, this is how to do it.

And the time is *right now.*

CHAPTER 2

WHY SHOULD YOU BECOME A HOLISTIC HEALTH PRACTITIONER?

"The paths most worn and used are also the most deceptive. So, nothing needs to be emphasized more than that we should not, like sheep, follow the lead of the flock in front of us—heading not where we ought to go, but where it goes."

Seneca, On the Happy Life

Much of modern education involves repetition, memorization, and regurgitation. And sadly, it's mostly theory. What if you, for example, have a burning desire to master the guitar? You probably won't take too many lessons from a teacher who only expounds on music theory. No, you will want to touch the guitar, learn a few chords, and start making music! That's the whole point: to make music.

Were you to become a holistic health practitioner, expect your training to be hands-on. If you pursue this field with my help, I will make sure you are not just interested in the theory—but in the practice. I will make sure that you understand what's going on, can affect a change, and are prepared to actually help someone, not just talk about it.

We don't graduate holistic health theorists; we graduate holistic health practitioners. That's a big difference.

So now you may ask: *why should I learn these skills and practices from Blue Lotus Institute for Holistic Studies?*

Knowing How to Help Someone

On one level, helping someone with their health seems easy. With some clients, you might recommend situational advice, like that they stop eating certain foods that are defeating them. That seems simple enough, right?

But you might move them to an area beyond just making a simple change, into helping them get their health under control and understand it on a much deeper level. Some people like to think they know everything about health when they only master one science, like yoga, aromatherapy, diet, or lifestyle. The truth is, it's a combination of every health art and science that moves someone to an area "beyond"—and that's what Blue Lotus Institute for Holistic Studies imparts.

For example, as a result of our program, you not only would be able to provide nutrition suggestions, but you may be equipped to help someone consistently digest food more easily. With the knowledge I share in our Institute, you will learn how to advise on specific practices that make a major difference, such as the many types of fasting—as well as cleanses.

Holistic health practitioners need to have *all* of this knowledge in their toolkits, because these practices actually move people in the right direction for their wellness. These are the tools you—and your clients—won't get just by studying theory or skimming the surface.

I also teach dinacharya in my practice, the Sanskrit word that means *daily lifestyle and habits supported by herbs.* Most practitioners think that dinacharya suggests you take herbs, for example, to improve your life. But it's the other way around. If you practice dinacharya, you live by its foundation—meaning you work on your whole life first, with the herbs being a component and complement. That means that you go to bed at the right time, think the right thoughts, and live by its principles. The herbs just make it easier. No, dinacharya is not just taking herbs, pulling oil, or boiling turmeric as the magical path to developing wellness. Dinacharya is a holistic practice, and I'll show you how to maximize it in your own life. You will learn to apply it for your own benefit first—and then the benefit of your clients and family members.

Understanding the Components of a Holistic Health Practitioner

Imagine if traditional doctors were schooled in Eastern, non-traditional, and holistic practices—as well as from Western medical textbooks! And imagine what more you could accomplish in your work if you incorporated the strongest components of holistic health.

Applying these practices, which I teach at our Institute, would be like a massage therapist having X-ray vision in their fingertips while working on a client. Instead of treating clients based on whatever was checked off on your menu of services, you would see the client's health in a whole new light.

A holistic health practitioner will observe more deeply and intuitively into their clients' needs as they take a holistic view of the body. Our Institute helps provide that X-ray level view into your holistic health.

Nurses love my Institute, since most of their training has come from one angle of medicine. They thirst to know more, because they know their background in allopathy isn't enough to help their clients. Many nurses have told me that they have bought several books on holistic health, but they can't put all of the pieces together. But when they come to my Institute, they become practitioners by following each module in a logical, sequential way.

Those who come to me with a medical background find themselves surprised at the host of holistic practices they've never even heard of—much less been exposed to, or taught how to apply.

Traditional medicine seeks to "cure" with a pill. Your head hearts? Here's a pill. You're feeling anxious? Here's another pill. You can't sleep? Guess what, another pill! You get the idea.

My Institute does give healers options outside of the pharmaceutical realm. I teach practitioners how to use natural remedies and natural substances, and I teach them dinacharya, a concept completely missed in allopathy. Imagine what would happen if patients turned away from big pharma and improved their wellness by examining and changing their daily lifestyle and habits! Imagine what you could do for your business if you worked in a health food store or vitamin shop, and you and your employees had this knowledge. Imagine what would happen if—instead of running to urgent care—you could help your family get better without a drug or M.D.?

I'm not saying that herbs cure everything. There is a time to go to a traditional medical practice. But for all those times in between—which is the majority of your life—the principles we teach will change the way you respond.

For a moment, put yourself in the position of someone who runs a vitamin shop. When someone comes in for help, do you listen? Do you understand where they're coming from? Are you able to ask questions related to causation to demonstrate that you know your stuff?

One practitioner told me of a customer who came to her vitamin shop saying, "I have pain, so I was thinking of trying turmeric."

Keep in mind, many of these well-intentioned customers went to Google to self-diagnose and prescribe. And it's great that they possess the awareness that they can't get every solution from a pill or medical office. But they still don't possess enough information to truly help themselves—and in some cases, their lack of knowledge or even misinformation may hurt them. Google is filtered with people's opinions and cluttered with allopathic/pharmaceutical belief. People want one pill—or even one herbal remedy—to cure everything; but the body doesn't work like that.

Instead of just pointing the customer to the turmeric options, the trained holistic health practitioner says, "Do you mind if I ask you a few questions so I can better guide you? Where is your pain exactly? Can you describe what the pain feels like? How are your bowels functioning?" And guess what? The customer doesn't need turmeric. She needs an excellent bowel formula, because her backache is a result of being backed up and storing toxins in her body.

Or perhaps, that practitioner could diagnose a customer with a sugar addiction by looking at their tongue and demeanor, and asking questions about their habits. Knowing the true problem, that practitioner could prescribe the right tonic or herbal remedy to get their customer onto a healthier path. Where do you think that customer would go next time they had a health need?

If you own a vitamin shop, wouldn't it be phenomenal if you not only sold supplements—but also greatly improved the lives of your customers with your newly-acquired experience? And if you don't own a vitamin shop, wouldn't it be life-changing if you held this knowledge yourself—even if just to assist your own family before ever setting foot into a medical office?

I also love working with chiropractors. It wasn't long ago that practitioners of chiropractic services were branded as witch doctors because of their unconventional practices. Chiropractors often have some level of awareness about nutrition, vitamins, and herbs, but these usually serve as secondary tools in their toolkit. For the most part, chiropractors practice common, standard processes and get effective results. But imagine what would happen if they increased their depth of understanding of holistic health practices!

For example, let me go back to how a good bowel movement can "eliminate" back pain by flushing out toxins. Many times, affecting a positive, long-term change for the chiropractic patient means treating bowels and parts of the lymphatic system.

Years ago when I had a problem with toxins, I would get a chiropractic adjustment, but nothing moved. Not only did adjustments hurt, but they wouldn't hold. I continually got out of adjustment. But once I learned how to clear my lymphatic system, my adjustments held. That's testament to the power of blending excellent chiropractic practices with real holistic health practices.

Schools and corporations often employ nurses to deal with day-to-day issues like headaches or stubbed toes. For the most part, these nurses don't have a wide range of tools at their disposal. Can you imagine if, in addition to traditional training, these nurses received experience as holistic health practitioners? Take any traditional healthcare practitioner, and add the right holistic health methodologies. Doing so doubles their effectiveness and tools available.

So why would you want to be a trained holistic health practitioner? First, it forces you to get your shit together (pun somewhat intended). Second, once you've gotten it together, you are qualified to help others find their way. I can tell you from my personal experience that this journey greatly improved my wellness and the wellness of those I serve.

Do you know the fine print in ads that says, "Individual results may vary"? All I can tell you is this: this holistic health practitioner journey changed my life when nothing else worked. It forced me to come to grips with myself and take that first long look in the mirror. Once I did that, I developed the skills and know-how required to address the things that weren't working for me. I learned how to handle things I didn't know how to handle before. It broadened my awareness and made me strive to perfect my daily practices.

If you're still on the fence, take heart. Several years ago, I would have been like, "Oh, hell, no. This is just a bunch of herbs, Ayurveda, and pseudo-spiritual nonsense." But then I started seeing results in my own life. I started to understand how I could make a real impact on the lives of others. As I furthered my studies and refined these courses, I learned what it takes to be a healer. Once I internalized and became a student of these best-practices, I set out to help others *get it* by simplifying and making the information accessible to as many people as possible.

If you're reading this and intuitively know that you have internal struggles or challenges with your well-being, I can show you a way to deal with it. Refuse to suffer through continual sugar cravings, insomnia, or stomach pains. Just because you've gotten used to being out of whack doesn't mean you have to stay that way. Let me show you how to heal yourself on your journey to helping others.

For Your Loved Ones

Lastly, the reason why you would want to be a holistic health practitioner is for your loved ones, which I've hinted at, but I haven't really explained it. Let's say your child wakes up screaming with a fever. You won't need to panic. Instead, you'll take his temperature and immediately know what herbs will provide him relief. In fact, once you're immersed in becoming a holistic health practitioner, you will develop a new, better way of life.

For example, when I go out to eat with friends, they know I'm going to start talking about the food. I'll say things like, "Oh, I see they have tabouli. That's great! Did you know it's full of parsley, which is an outstanding natural diuretic?" I don't need to sound like an annoying know-it-all, because I share in a way that is so natural and authentic, who wouldn't want to learn more? You will view your new way of life as something you can't wait to share with others, and those around you will benefit from how you connect food and daily activities as a way to promote natural healing.

Ayurveda teaches us that all diseases start from one of two ways: the misuse of our senses or mistake of our intellect. When you're ready to be the change you wish to see in the world, you will activate your senses and improve your intellect. When you choose to expand your knowledge and skills as a certified holistic health practitioner through Blue Lotus Institute for Holistic Studies, or come to Blue Lotus Healing Center (which is the side of our business that focuses on providing care to clients), you'll enter a world that forever changes how you react to circumstances, how you view the world, and you deal with disease.

CHAPTER 3

WHERE TO START

"Health seeks health. Unhealthy seeks unhealthy. Energy seeks itself."

David D. Jameson, DNM

Doctor of Natural Medicine

If you're considering getting into the healing arts, or if you're already in the healing arts and want to add Certified Holistic Health Practitioner to your repertoire, know that all holistic health practitioner research will lead you back to Blue Lotus Institute for Holistic Studies. You've heard that "all roads lead to Rome"? Well, all serious research about becoming a holistic health practitioner will lead you back to our site for information. We are that good, and for the right reasons.

But you don't have to take my word for it. First off, do your homework. I recommend that you make a list of things you want to research about holistic health and various institutes. For example, here are some questions I recommend you research or ask:

- How do they define a *holistic health practitioner*?
- What is included in their curriculum?
- What do others have to say about them? What is their reputation?

Consider reading five or six general articles about the work of holistic health practitioners. It won't be long before you find Blue Lotus Institute for Holistic Studies. Then research several different institutes. Compare the curriculum carefully, because you will find some significant differences.

Fairly quickly, you'll understand that even the definition of holistic health practitioner varies from institute to institute. I've had people come into my clinic and proudly hand me a card with *holistic health practitioner* embossed on it. I'm like, "What? What do you do?" I mean, that title could mean anything. They could be a gardener or a Reiki master. That's how loose of a term *holistic health practitioner* is in general use.

And I have to say that it bothers me, because the people who work really hard to get this designation *deserve* that designation. It must have meaning behind it! That's why we're constantly working on our affiliations to provide you with even more leverage in the broader world. Blue Lotus Institute for Holistic Studies is broadening our relationship with groups like the American Association of Drugless Practitioners, to make membership simpler and more streamlined—and certifications accredited. We are working with major universities, like the University of Natural Medicine, to integrate and collaborate with their doctoral programs. If you're working on a naturopath doctorate or a doctor of natural medicine like I did, or even a PhD, you likely want a program that complements it, rather than competes with it—or worse yet, seems to exist in a vacuum. Our future collaborations are promising, because we are the best. Read what the masses have to say about us. The reputation of where you study matters greatly. And ask us for the latest updates on our collaborations and accreditations, because most likely, progress will have been made after this book is printed. We are agile and always improving the service and value we offer to our students.

Once you've researched various holistic health institutes, I'm sure you'll agree that Blue Lotus Institute for Holistic Studies stands heads and shoulders above the rest. I've sequenced our program to walk people through a groundwork of what follows; it's not purely theoretical. Of course we teach theory, but our process ensures that we aren't graduating mere theorists but rather practitioners.

Look at what graduates from other institutes do with their certificates. What kind of work do they perform? We try to align your desired objectives with practical training, so when you finish, you are prepared to do your most meaningful work ever. If you're looking to practice or obtain a deeper knowledge of how to help people, you won't find anything better than Blue Lotus Institute for Holistic Studies.

One huge differentiator of our programs is how we lay the foundation for learning. For example, let's say a student doesn't have a background in Ayurveda. Instead of training you in depth in Ayurveda, we will make sure you understand the basics of Ayurveda processes so you can reap the rewards. It's like if you want to learn to fish. Do you really need to read several books on the history of fishing in North America? No! You need the basics: a rod, reel, hook, and some bait. Our framework gives you enough knowledge to start helping others. Let's say you have a client with digestive issues and toxins built up. Most naturopaths have enough knowledge to ask questions, or possibly order a blood test. In other words, they have enough knowledge to chase symptoms. Our real-world instruction gives you several additional tools and a broader knowledge base to treat the causes, not just the symptoms.

After you have received a good foundation from our program, you will learn how to work on subtle energies. You will learn how to uncover causation—where things are coming from. Chasing symptoms is easy. Any worker at a health food store or CVS can give you something for your backache. But can they help you get to the root of the problem? That's the difference between well-intended individuals with limited knowledge—and what you would receive from the best holistic health practitioner.

You already know that back aches could be caused from any number of things. Maybe it's an overworked muscle. It could be that the lymph is in misalignment. Perhaps it's a problem with digestion or stemming from the kidneys. Without a system, you chase a symptom; however, with a symptom **and** a system, you can find causation.

Blue Lotus Institute for Holistic Studies is the only program that offers such a robust framework. For example, we use Ayurveda. Not even traditional Chinese medicine offers a framework as strong as Ayurveda.

In short, too many educational institutes stay in the world of theories. Not us. We graduate holistic health **practitioners**, not holistic health educators or holistic health technicians. We want to send you back to your community equipped to practice, not theorize!

CHAPTER 4

GOOD OR BAD REP

"If you want to flow down the river of health you have to let go of the branch of fear."

David D. Jameson, DNM

Doctor of Natural Medicine

We all know society prefers the herd mentality. Right now, you have people that can't even explain what's going on in society, but they will argue with you because they prefer to be part of the herd, and they don't want to stray from the masses.

This applies to holistic medicine, too. Does it have a good reputation or a bad one? Instead of following the herd and listening to the traditional, indoctrinated masses in Western healthcare, understand that what others think about holistic health is based on their perceptions.

Several years ago, the American Medical Association and Big Pharma got behind a documentary about chiropractic medicine. It was a hatchet job! The movie skewered chiropractic medicine and started saying and repeating a mantra over and over again:

"Chiropractors aren't real doctors!" That false narrative became embedded in the minds of many people, and even though it's false, many came to accept it as truth. All of this criticism just because doctors of chiropractic medicine didn't want to march a goosestep with traditional allopathic physicians. But they are still physicians! I'm a doctor of natural medicine. Just because I don't write prescriptions for benzos, anti-depressants, and addictive, pain-numbing narcotics doesn't mean I'm not a physician!

Isn't this the same group of medical experts who refused to say that cigarette smoking created health problems for many years? Isn't this the same group of medical experts who tell us that PSA, the prostate-specific antigen, is a marker for cancer? Yet I've personally interviewed Dr. Richard Ablin, a scientist from University of Arizona College of Medicine, who along with colleagues discovered PSA, leading to the PSA test. He told me it should not be relied on for routine screening (to get the details as he puts them, see his book, *The Great Prostate Hoax: How Big Medicine Hijacked the PSA Test and Caused a Public Health Disaster, which he* co authored with Richard Albin, 2014)! In other words, consider the source as you form your own opinions and perceptions about any branch of science. From where I stand, modern medicine works best when coupled with holistic health practices. The two can and should work together, instead of being at odds.

Some traditional health practitioners want to leave the security of their herds, but they are too afraid to do so. The truth is, they don't have to leave traditional medicine; however, they could certainly benefit by broadening their knowledge bases.

We holistic health practitioners understand that bodies are bombarded regularly with an assortment of toxic chemicals that wreak havoc on livers and bowels. Instead of using traditional medicine alone (where they treat the symptoms, remember?), people could benefit from the knowledge of a holistic health practitioner. While traditional medicine can offer short-term relief of symptoms, a holistic health practitioner could help the client lower blood sugar levels naturally through creating a better diet and healthier lifestyle plan. The two disciplines can work in support of one another.

Too often, though, both sides overstep their boundaries. Allopathy claims to offer "health care." In reality, there is no health care. There is symptom care.

Physicians write prescriptions for medications with no plan to wean people off those medicines, perhaps having convinced themselves that "they haven't died yet, so this seems to be working." Then they never talk with the patient about making needed dietary and lifestyle changes that will actually improve health and resolve the problem. Too many doctors follow these "protocols," because it's lucrative and certainly much easier than having a tough, time-consuming conversation with a possibly resistant patient.

Additionally, even amongst doctors wanting to point the patient towards improved health, few doctors have the knowledge.

Granted, sadly, some holistic health practitioners and holistic doctors overstep their boundaries, trying to affect cures in advanced diseases. While we can treat many ailments, we can't cure the incurable. Besides, many cures rest more with the client than with the practitioner.

Yes, both traditional medicine and holistic medicine step over the line at times by venturing into areas where they are outside of the expertise. Both require ongoing discretion—and learning.

From my own experience as a doctor of natural medicine, I've had people walk into my office after seeing another naturopathic doctor. I've looked over my colleague's protocols. After seeing several people who first visited another naturopathic doctor, something occurred to me: all of the people were given the same diet. I couldn't believe it! We are unique individuals, and our bodies have different needs. How could they all possibly be put on the same diet?

I learned from that experience how important the right training and the absence of bias is in our work. An elderly priest and an adolescent female might both see a doctor for acne. A trained holistic health practitioner would see if these individuals had a sugar addiction. They would adjust their diets and lifestyles, understanding that these are unique individuals. But if a teenage girl with acne visits an allopathic practitioner, that doctor would say, "I think we need to put you on birth control." So now the doctor has messed with her hormones, when the cause is most likely lymphatic.

The manifestation of matter starts with consciousness, easily demonstrated through multiple personality disorders (MPD) and hypnotism. Let's say Jim has dissociative identity disorder (DID), what used to be known as multiple personality disorder. Jim is addicted to cigarettes and nicotine. He's also on insulin, because his pancreas isn't functioning correctly. But when another personality, let's say Bill, takes over his body, everything changes. Bill hates cigarettes; the smell drives him crazy. Something else happens when Jim becomes Bill: Bill's pancreas works fine. Same tissue, same organism, same person, but completely different body functioning! Perception informs reality.

It's true of hypnotism, too. When we enter a state where we are susceptible to suggestion, it changes our behaviors and perception of reality.

You have probably heard of the placebo effect. If we could put the placebo effect into a pill, that would be one worth taking! But of course, we can't, because it exists in the power of the mind. What we can do is help people tap into the power of their minds to influence health. Numerous podcasts detail this phenomenon, because it's so powerful. What we believe to be true can become reality.

Again, *it's more important to know what kind of patient has a disease, than what kind of disease the patient has*. By treating the person—including helping with their mindset—we can help them heal.

Joining the Holistic Health Practitioner Certification Program at Blue Lotus Institute for Holistic Studies teaches you to leave your assumptions at the door and meet people where they are. It doesn't matter if those you help are using allopathic medicines or anything like that; you can still help them. Holistic health practitioners treat people who are ready to change for the better, ready to turn things around. Holistic health practitioners have the training to provide the best possible remedies for a host of issues and people.

CHAPTER 5

THE DECISION

"Natural medicine heals your life."

David D. Jameson, DNM

Doctor of Natural Medicine

As I stated earlier, when you come to our Certified Holistic Health Practitioner program at Blue Lotus Institute for Holistic Studies, the first thing you will confront is how you might be making mistakes in your thinking. You must tackle your own issues before you have the credibility and experience to help others.

Now I want to share with you the structure of our modules in the Blue Lotus Institute for Holistic Studies Certified Holistic Health Practitioner program. (At any time, feel free to learn more on our website, (www.bluelotushealingcenter.com).

Module One: Foundations—Ecology & Spirit, and Introduction to Ayurveda

Module One covers our Foundations: Ecology & Spirit, and Introduction to Ayurveda. We start with the book *In Search of the Medicine Buddha*, by David Crow, a doctor who shares his experiences as he traveled across India. He shares about how his American way of thinking about medicine was all wrong. For example, he discusses minerals and toxic metals, and myths about them that, when unraveled, hold keys to healing. This book sets the stage for everything you will learn, in that it teaches you to question truths and mistruths you've taken for granted. When I first read this book, I was blown away. That's all I will say about it except this: the book changed my life.

In that same module, you will learn about the ancient teaching of Ayurveda—and how to bring its principles into the *now*. Remember, our program gives you groundwork—a framework in which to work. The reason Ayurveda works so well in our program is because you don't have to be an Ayurvedic practitioner or an Ayurvedic doctor to understand and apply the principles.

The principles and a framework are what help you become more than strictly a symptom treater. Treating symptoms alone obviously doesn't work. If it did, we would be the healthiest nation in the world.

Module Two: The Building Blocks—Aroma 101

Module Two is The Building Blocks, which covers Aroma 101. Not surprisingly, this part of the program focuses on the power of aromatherapy. Right at this moment, some of you may have a thought pop into your head: "Aromatherapy? Gadzooks! That's hocus pocus at best!" Here's why I love aromatherapy. Let's say you walk next to a blossoming apple tree. Obviously, the tree doesn't say anything to you as you walk by. But communication is still taking place. On an almost subconscious level, you may recognize that smell as one that reminds you of playing at your grandmother's house when you were a child. Poof! That sensory memory is a hint that there's something holographic being stored in your body. When you can affect that change in your mood based on an olfactory response, then it doesn't really matter where it's coming from, if it's a change from within. Ironically, many of the people who enter the aromatherapy class cynical end up reporting that it's one of their favorite classes. Learn how to assess the quality of essential oils—and channel the energy of aroma!

Module Three: Herbal Medicine

Module Three is all about Herbal Medicine. While it's an introductory course, it still goes into quite a lot of depth. You'll learn about lymphatic bowel health, how to help people with anxiety and other types of stress, adaptogens like immunomodulators, and how to keep people at their optimum health. This module contains the most helpful information about plants, tinctures, powdered formulas, and dosages. If an herb serves a known medicinal purpose, you will learn about it in this module.

Module Four: The Pathways—An Introduction to Homeopathy, Digestion, and Diet & Lifestyle

Module Four, The Pathways, includes three sections. The first is An Introduction to Homeopathy, which covers the full gamut of homeopathic medicine. The second focuses on Digestion. And the final section digs into the key to good health: Diet & Lifestyle.

By the time you get into Module Four, you will start working with clients in a real-world setting. Homeopathy is a wonderful way to have a vast array of herbs without having a giant apothecary. I have an apothecary at our healing center that takes up around eight hundred square feet. If it's a healing herb, I own and maintain it. That's how I have learned so much about how these herbs work, and it's how I offer the best insight to my students—and best treatment to my clients. During your time studying through the Institute, you will learn all the best practices from age-old wisdom—and modern practices, including my own experience.

As a holistic health practitioner, you will have access to all of the basic homeopathic remedies to help people with colds, fevers, and other common ailments. But at the beginning of working with someone (or yourself), because Ayurveda is all about digestion and elimination and state of the body, we have to ask if our body and tissues are functioning correctly or incorrectly before taking the next steps.

By the time you learn about diet and exercise, you'll be ready to discover how to promote healthy lifestyle changes that stick. You will learn about juicing, fasting, and seasonal cleansing—and how to sustain a healthy diet lifestyle. Remember dinacharya, the Sanskrit concept I mentioned earlier? Herbs support diet and a healthy lifestyle. We'll teach you how to integrate these elements. We'll also teach you why you can't live a junk diet lifestyle and overwrite the ill effects by taking dandelion root! A diet lifestyle is very important for helping someone effect a change and meet their health goals.

The Specialization Project

As part of your program, we offer this unique opportunity to focus in more depth on a specific area of interest, such as: Herbology, Ayurveda, Aromatherapy and/or Whole Food Nutrition.

Instead of this module having pre-developed coursework, we allow you to submit a question or topic you would most like to learn more about. Then we help you find the resources to develop your expertise in that area. For me, when I was a student at the Institute (before I was the owner and operator), I chose to use my Specialization Project to learn more about all things holistic.

Have I piqued your intrigue in these topics? Are you ready to satiate that curiosity with more knowledge? It's time! If you want to experience a new level of health—and help others do the same—you've got to be ready to effect a change within yourself. Some members of the herd might give you strange looks. Let them. Clients wanting relief and ready to take ownership of their health like never before will see you differently, because you will know things that others find a mystery.

In no time, you'll be receiving the rewards of clients (and family members!) calling you just to say they are feeling better, that they've turned their health issues around, and that they credit your help with making the biggest difference.

CHAPTER 6

HOLISTIC MEDICINE PAST

"If the lymph isn't right, nothing will be right."

David D. Jameson

Doctor of Natural Medicine

It wasn't long ago when we didn't use labels like *holistic* or *alternative*. It was just *medicine*. And we didn't call those health care providers "doctor"; we called them Grandma!

Grandma cooked recipes passed down from generations that contained real foods (not full of additives and chemicals)—healing foods. Grandma wouldn't dream of eating or serving her family fast food or junk food. No, instead, Grandma would make soup in the winter—and light, easily-digestible foods in the summer—cooking whatever vegetables happened to be in season to ensure they still contained all of the natural nutrients that God intended. When Grandma noticed that little Johnny seemed off, caught the sniffles, or became constipated, Grandma knew what teas and herbs would aid his digestion.

Grandparents taught their children these timeless remedies, and then those children passed the secrets down to their own children. That's the way medicine worked. And it was effective.

Yet the American Medical Association would have us believe that those remedies don't work—that "real" medicine must use lab-created chemicals and pharmaceutical solutions instead. Why? Follow the money! Big Pharma spends billions of dollars each year courting doctors to show off the latest and greatest pill for whatever ails you.

Allopathy would say, "Okay, you say your quackery works? What would you give someone with cancer? How would you cure someone of cancer?" Seriously? It doesn't work like that. The grandparents took care of the kids. Their knowledge was passed on to the next generation. And so on.

And it was effective. A medical system that says otherwise is misleading you. It worked very well, if you use it as a lifestyle.

Holistic medicine works when it's part of a lifestyle. Can it cure cancer? No. But can it help your body function in its optimal state to help prevent cancer? Absolutely.

As you learn more about holistic medicine, your eyes may be opened—even to the way you've learned history. For example, I even wonder if so-called witches from the Salem witch trials were actually herbalists. These individuals could cure with potions and herbs. But herbalists' practices threatened traditional doctors who used "science" to cure instead of ancient remedies. These traditional doctors knew, for example, that when you were treating someone with an acute throat infection or pneumonia, the best treatment involved letting out all of the bad blood.

Do you know what killed George Washington? His doctor drained nearly 40 percent of Washington's blood to "cure" his throat infection. Frankly, I believe that an herbalist would have treated his infection more effectively.

An ancient Chinese proverb says this about holistic medicine: "The doctor gets paid when the village is well." What a refreshing paradigm!

Western medicine takes the opposite approach, one that seems to practice, "My path to riches is for you to stay sick!" Ironically, even traditional medical practitioners have started to see the benefits of "hippie fringe" concepts like kombucha and probiotics as part of improving overall health. Isn't it interesting that a focus on creating a healthy biome in our guts has been part of holistic health from time immemorial? The AMA now invests money conducting clinical trials of fecal transplants as a way of recreating healthy gut biomes. But we holistic health practitioners know how to help our clients foster and maintain a healthy gut through healthy diet, nutrition, and habits.

Thomas Edison famously predicted that "the doctor of the future will no longer treat the human frame with drugs, but rather will cure and prevent disease with nutrition." The future is now, and it's called holistic health!

Modern life grows more fast-paced and complicated each day, driving sick folks to seek quick, simple fixes for anything that's wrong with them. Today, we have more chemicals in our foods and in the air we breathe than ever before. We have more stress. Our thirty-hour work week increased to forty, then fifty, and now some people work sixty-plus hours each week just to pay the bills. Fewer families believe they can make a living on one paycheck, so dual income families are the norm. With all of this stress pressing down, it's no wonder that few people have the patience for Grandma's natural, lifestyle-centered medicine.

Sadly, though, allopathic medicine can come with a great cost to your long-term health, and without Grandma's lifestyle practices, poor health will return.

Big Pharma and Quick Fixes

One of the biggest challenges to the proven efficacy of holistic health practices is the money that flows from Big Pharma into allopathy. Big Pharma can't make money on holistic remedies and treatments. When the AMA and Big Pharma decide to test a holistic remedy, they conduct those tests in a vacuum and then claim, "We couldn't find evidence that this treatment did anything beneficial."

Heck, no treatment will be effective if it's administered incorrectly! Let's say they want to test the efficacy of turmeric on someone with a toxic lymphatic system. Yes, turmeric DOES reduce inflammation. But it won't work if that guy goes home and drinks a quart of gin and eats a pint of ice cream each night! Selective tests on holistic remedies conducted by Western medicine don't have rigorous controls or include lifestyle changes as part of the testing. No doctor of natural medicine or holistic health practitioner claims that any magical herb or natural treatment can override an unhealthy lifestyle.

No wonder so many sick people want the easy cure! They've been led to believe that their poor health has nothing to do with their own unhealthy behaviors. So when a doctor offers to treat the symptoms, too many people believe that allopathy cures disease. But by now you know that it doesn't cure disease as much as it treats symptoms.

Learning Beyond the Classroom

I've found that where you've gone to school and received your training is of great importance to most people. But sometimes it doesn't lead to the most well-rounded or forward-thinking person. Have you ever met someone who graduated from a top school yet didn't have the sense to open the umbrella tucked under his arm during a downpour? Or have you ever met someone who never finished school yet possessed more insight and intuition than anyone you've ever met? It's not just about where you go to school: it's about the results you achieve.

Before my dean signed my doctorate diploma, he requested that I send forty files from differing individuals to him. Forty! Do you know what he did with those files?

He made sure that the people I treated saw health improvements as a result of my work. As he handed me my diploma, he told me that he had learned so much from me. Me, a student! And he told me I had been doing a fantastic job. I don't bring this up to brag. Rather, I want you to understand that what I learned and now practice didn't come only from an institute or some professors with long designations after their names. No, instead I learned from anyone I could, taking courses all over the spectrum, acquiring the skills I could use to help people get better. That's what the Blue Lotus Institute for Holistic Studies HHP program does for wellness. I took the long route to learning.

Today, I take what I learned on my journey, distill it down to the core basics, and offer it to you.

Becoming a holistic health practitioner isn't a "once and done" sort of thing. It's not an event. It's about becoming a life-long student where your study never ends. It's about staying current on the latest research as a way of offering the broadest range of remedies. For example, at my clinic, Blue Lotus Healing Center, we have frequency generators like PEMF (pulsed electromagnetic field), because I've found that that's where all energy comes from: frequency and voltage. PEMF is necessary if you want to live. No joke. NASA figured this out when they sent astronauts into space, and they came back extremely ill. They had everything they needed, they thought: food, water, shelter, so why were they so violently ill? The astronauts were slowly getting better after returning to Earth, so NASA figured that space had to be lacking something. The answer was simple: PEMF. After a four-year study, NASA confirmed that PEMF has extraordinary benefits. PEMF machines work in conjunction with the body's own recovery process to alleviate pain by restoring the cells' ability to function properly. Our specific PEMF machine at Blue Lotus Healing Center has a magnetic impulse generator which gives the Schumann frequencies during the therapy, which is considered the heartbeat of the Earth, vibrating at 7.83 hertz. Our bodies need electricity to send signals to the brain and other parts of the body to function properly. PEMF therapy effectively realigns the electric potential of the cells. Simply put, without PEMF, we die.

We are connected to this energy through nature. Nature gives us these frequencies when we ground our feet in the dirt. So, when we're trapped in buildings, driving in cars with rubber tires, wearing shoes with rubber soles, and surrounded by Wi-Fi routers and 5G towers, these PEMF signals are blocked, slowly depleting our health.

We will remain thirsty for any viable treatment options that become available, but we will never eschew the lessons passed on from generations that our grandmothers knew.

I am sure you've heard the phrases, "Everything old is new again," and, "There is nothing new under the sun." That's especially true in the healing arts.

Before aspirin, man used the leaves from the willow tree for 2,400 years. What is aspirin? It's man's attempt to copy and improve medicine that's been around since before Christ.

For more than 4,000 years, licorice root was used as a curative for asthma. Today, we know licorice root contains glycyrrhizin, a powerful antiviral, with anti-inflammatory properties as well as a natural way to relieve symptoms of IBS and Crohn's disease.

As I tell my holistic health practitioner students, don't confuse new with better. It turns out, Grandma could teach those in allopathy a few things.

CHAPTER 7

THE FUTURE OF HOLISTIC MEDICINE

"It is a paradox that to get healthy, you must be healthy. The word Dinacharya means appropriate daily lifestyle and habits. Dinacharya is the cornerstone of Ayurveda and places us in the vibrational frequency that allows nature to do its healing work... thus telling the Universe, 'I am healthy.' Wanting to be healthy affirms lack. Proper Dinacharya affirms health."

David D. Jameson, DNM
Doctor of Natural Medicine

Sixty years ago, could you imagine that one day we'd be seeing a TV commercial or an advertisement in a magazine enticing consumers to take a new miracle treatment for eczema, plaque psoriasis, or gingivitis? And in that same ad, either via voice-over or in the very fine print, that you'd find a warning that this treatment could cause *anal seepage, hair loss, nausea, impotence, infertility, suicidal ideation, cancer, constipation, depression, diarrhea, drowsiness, dizziness, distemper, dry mouth, dermatitis, or death?*

What changed? Big Pharma started marketing directly to consumers, taking control of the most profitable segment of healthcare, and wormed its way into everyone's lives. "Ask your doctor if _______ is right for you." Isn't that what the ads say? So in the rare occasion that your provider isn't already incented to write you a prescription for the "latest and greatest" medication, Big Pharma wants consumers to suggest their medications to their care providers.

Sadly, people often believe these massive PR machines when these companies with ulterior motives convince the world that they are offering the most intelligent, best, and most scientifically advanced formula ever. And even more sadly for consumers, Big Pharma spends millions each year attacking non-traditional medical practices.

Let me ask you this: if Big Pharma offers the most intelligent, best, and most scientifically advanced treatments, why would they bother to take the time and money to put down its so-called competition? Isn't that funny? No, it's sad. Follow the money. Big Pharma exists to make new drugs to generate more revenue, and they feel threatened if even a pittance of healthcare dollars go anywhere except in their big pockets.

The AMA and most medical schools stand alongside Big Pharma. Do you remember what I wrote earlier about the AMA's slandering of chiropractic medicine? In the documentary, *Doctored,* the AMA goes after chiropractic treatment as if it were a venomous, seven-headed snake. Why would the AMA go after chiropractors? Follow the money. The AMA needs you to stay sick, because healthy people don't generate revenue.

I can't tell you how many allopathic medical students have told me that they were given shiny print propaganda putting down herbs, homeopathy, and chiropractic services—while they were still in med school. If the AMA were a cult, we'd call that brainwashing. In order for traditional medicine to grow, it needs to secure followers and adherents as soon as they enter medical school.

It's gotten to the point where I dislike the labels "traditional" or "non-traditional" medicine, because they are misleading. In fact, they seem backwards. As I shared in the previous chapter, thousands of years ago, man used willow leaves for the same curative effect as aspirin. Shouldn't we call willow leaves *traditional* and *natural*, whereas aspirin is *non-traditional, synthetic,* and *unnatural*?

The medicine men of old, or the so-called witch doctors, used herbs to promote healing and health. Their treatments worked. These traditional healers did not go to a diagnostic manual or use a pull-down menu to select a drug protocol for treatment. Rather, they listened carefully to the people they were treating

. They asked questions to better understand the cause of their ailments. And they practiced non-invasive healing, including tinctures.

But in the allopathic mind, holistic medicine is seen as a threat to wellness. Really? That's like an elephant feeling threatened by a dung beetle. Big Pharma and the AMA possess all the power and money.

Holistic medicine, at its worst, doesn't solve every person's problems. But it helps people live better lives. Why would the FDA ban homeopathy? The worst that can happen if someone takes too many or the wrong herbs is an upset stomach. It's nearly impossible to harm someone deeply and permanently with herbs.

Can allopathic practitioners say that about even such "safe" and "proven" over-the-counter medications like acetaminophen?

When people say we live in a "woke" society, they refer to a growing awareness around social and racial justice. But there's another awakening taking place, one where people have become "woke" to the energetic side of healing and well-being.

Some people have referred to me as a Reiki master. But isn't everybody? Don't we all possess at least some ability to serve as chronic healers? Holistic health practitioners learn how to tap into all the senses to observe sickness, proffer solutions, and bring about healthier lifestyles. As more people become "woke" to the power of holistic practices, the less grip the elephants of Big Pharma, the AMA, and medical schools have over our health and well-being.

How do I know that an awakening is taking place? I've noticed an uptick in the number of vitamin shops, health food stores, chiropractic services, and healthful eateries featuring vegetarian and vegan options. The idea has finally broken into our collective consciousness that we can't jam unhealthy foods down our pie holes and expect improved health.

Likewise, people have caught on that healthful foods form the backbone of a healthy lifestyle. When we eat better, we feel better. As more people understand the power of our own energy, the more they demand access to fresh, healthful foods—and herbs and supplements.

Being a holistic health practitioner allows you to direct people away from the old paradigm that we've been sold, the one that says, "Every time you eat ______, you develop terrible reflux and heartburn. Take this pill thirty minutes before eating ______, so you can keep eating the things that make you feel like death!"

As a holistic health practitioner, you can identify what's wrong with this picture. When people experience gastric distress, you can direct them to ginger and peppermint instead of Zantac™ (removed from the market by the FDA in April 2020 for containing high levels of NDMA, a probable human carcinogen) or Pepcid AC™. Strange, I never remember a ginger tea recall due to it containing carcinogens or any other deadly substance.

Through natural, holistic remedies, you'll gain insight about educating people on what to do *instead* of reaching for a prescribed or OTC medication. You will hold the credibility and ability to teach those ready to make a change how to maintain well-being and health the natural way—fostering a better lifestyle.

Our minds are powerful creators. Just like the negative spin and outright slander from the mainstream medical community around holistic healing, I guarantee you that if the news told you tonight that COVID-19 causes blindness and vomiting, we would see millions of newly-"blind" people throwing up across the country tomorrow. That's the power of suggestion. It's real, and works like mass hypnotism.

So what can we holistic health practitioners do to combat that? We need more people to educate themselves and share what they've learned.

At the end of our certification program, I want you to be able to talk about holistic medicine from your own experience. Tell the success stories you've witnessed firsthand.

How about this one? A dual-credentialed M.D./N.D. had an elderly client visit her, asking if she would help him die. He was done living, exhausted from feeling so weak and sick all the time. After a conversation with the man, the doctor said, "Well, if you really think that you are ready for hospice care, how about we look at the medications you're currently taking. Some medications have such dreadful side effects that can make you feel as sick or sicker than the illness they are meant to treat." Guess what? The man had been prescribed twenty-two different medications, many of which were prescribed to counter the side effects of the other medications! By the end of the visit, the two of them agreed that he would stop taking eighteen of those medications. He came back the next week. Do you know what he reported? He felt better than he had felt in years. A month later, he felt better still. By the third month, the doctor did a complete blood workup. His results were better than any other lab work recorded over the last five years! Imagine if that doctor had just agreed to let the man die. Her patient didn't need another prescription. He needed to return his body to a state where it could use its energy to heal itself from the inside out.

Sometimes the opposing holistic health practitioners come from the inside. Not long ago, an Ayurvedic college contacted me, asking me to sit on their board.

"Let me ask you this," I said. "Do you practice traditional Ayurveda? Does your school base its teaching on the ancient texts?

The college dean stammered a moment, and then said, "Well, of course not. Those ancient texts are old. I mean really old. Besides, what happened in India thousands of years ago has little bearing on today. Instead of pulling out the old texts, we encourage people to practice Ayurveda the way they best see fit."

Sadly, that's not what those "really old" texts tell us—that these methods don't stand the test of time. The texts are very clear. Why would we want to dilute something that is so pure?

But I can't say that I'm surprised to see so-called Ayurvedic doctors moving away from Ayurvedic teachings. In fact, that started happening in India a hundred years ago. I know of Ayurveda practitioners with a Bachelor's of Ayurveda Medicine and Surgery (BAMS) degrees who don't practice traditional Ayurveda. I got a call recently from a BAMS doctor in India who wanted to know how he should treat someone with rheumatoid arthritis. Arthritis. Really? Have we moved so far away from the ancient wisdom that we don't know how to help with arthritis?

Even a study sponsored by the World Health Organization concluded that Ayurvedic treatment of rheumatoid arthritis showed "statistically significant improvement in all parameters [of rheumatoid arthritis patients] from admission to discharge." (https://www.ncbi.nlm.nih.gov/pmc/articles/PMC3157120/). Yet a degreed, credentialed Ayurvedic doctor from India, the birthplace of Ayurveda, had no idea how he could help.

That's why I stick to the ancient texts: they have withstood the test of time and proven their efficacy.

More significant than this Ayurvedic doctor not knowing the treatment protocols, how in the world could I lay out any treatment protocols knowing nothing about his patient's mental state, sleep patterns, or diet? I thought to myself, *This is crazy. I don't know anything about his patient, but you want me to commit to a treatment protocol?* Pretty nutty.

My holistic health practitioner program doesn't work like that at all. We aren't built around theories, and we don't offer one-size-fits-all treatments. What we do is based on the individual we are treating—and stems from a deep and broad knowledge-base that we unapologetically teach our practitioners.

That's what I mean about we, as practitioners, facing opposition from within. What we offer is different from what you will get elsewhere, in that we give you the fundamentals rooted in age-old truth, and we will help you think on your feet to apply what works best. When you mix truth with lies, you no longer have truth. Likewise, we can't water down proven, best-practices with "do as you see fit" philosophy—and claim we offer holistic health services.

Before you earn the designation of Certified Holistic Health Practitioner through the Blue Lotus Institute for Holistic Studies, you must be grounded in the universal facts that have been around for millennia. My training gives you confidence and know-how to serve as a healer.

The title of this chapter is "The Future of Holistic Medicine." So are you wondering why I spent so much time on the past? We must know the adversaries we face, as we bring new awareness about the ancient—as well as new—healing practices that encompass holistic health. We face deep-pocketed opponents whose very livelihoods depend on maintaining the status quo. We also face challenges from within by some of our own who would dilute our practices, often to the detriment of those we serve. But as far as the future of holistic medicine, we are in the middle of a great awakening. People are thinking for themselves, no longer content to let Big Pharma "heal" them. People understand that wellness is an inside job, and there is a new awareness that wellness is about lifestyle choices and options.

So for the holistic health practitioner, the future is bright. The world needs what we offer. And how we offer those services is limited only by our will to find—and apply—the truth.

CHAPTER 8

SCOPE OF PRACTICE

"We are spirits, in the material world."

The Police

People who wish to join the ranks of holistic health practitioner come from one of four backgrounds or drivers. Some people start with one objective, but along the way, they decide to do more—or less—with their education. Nearly all have one goal: to be better healers.

Driver #1: The Professional Holistic Health Practitioner

As the name suggests, these people desire to turn this education into their vocation. Some are already members of the healing arts, but they want to expand their repertoire. These folks want to know as much as possible, so they can take their healing to the next level with clients.

Driver #2: The Intellectually Curious

Some come to our Institute not looking to turn healing into a career. Instead, these people come because they have a passion to learn new things, perspectives, and a way of living. Fueled by intellectual curiosity, these passionate individuals want to expand their knowledge and pick up some useful remedies they can use at home.

Driver #3: The Professional Hobbyist

I have a lot of hobbies, mostly around learning and improving myself. One of my quirks is, I love to learn more about aliens. And with the news that UFOs are now accepted as reality even by our government, maybe that's not such a quirky interest anymore! I also love reading books, watching baseball, teaching important lessons to my kids, and practicing freedom of any kind.

We've graduated people from the Institute that thirst to learn about health and wellness, because it's like a professional hobby for them. They read anything they can get their hands on. They want to add even more knowledge, just like I don't watch the same baseball game over and over again. I move on to the next game, following the stats along the way. Professional hobbyists become fascinated by acquiring new knowledge around health-related subjects. As a side benefit, their hobby helps them personally, and helps their loved ones.

Driver #4: The Heart of a Healer

Finally, some people pursue becoming a holistic health practitioner so they can best nurture their loved ones. These people have no intention of profiting from this learning. They simply want to improve the health of those they love. Frankly, these make some of the best students.

Regardless of what stirred your desire to study holistic health, I promise you a rewarding journey. Maybe there are parts of your life that you've tried changing before, but you just couldn't manage to make positive changes stick. Perhaps something is sapping your mental and physical health, and you want to find a better way to live. I'll help you dig deep inside. I'll help you take that journey within, so you can see it, understand it, and deal with it in your own life. Then I'll show you how to remove any imbalance and free yourself to move forward. Once you've done that, you'll learn how to best help others.

If you're not convinced yet, let me share what I experienced in the Blue Lotus Institute for Holistic Studies Certified Holistic Health program before I purchased the center to run myself—and what others validated with no prompting from me. Here is what I've gained:

- **Empowerment.** That's the first thing I experienced when I started down this path. I felt empowered. I no longer had to rely on doctors with limited knowledge. I didn't need to consume pharmaceuticals to treat symptoms. Finally, I had the means to manage my health.

- **Accountability.** What I learned helped me take accountability for my own health. I learned to manage cravings and diet—on my own, without someone standing over me.

- **Confidence.** I developed the confidence to confront my own health issues and those of others. For the first time, I understood how the complex system that is the body actually works.

- **Weight loss and breaking addictions.** I lost weight, because the program forced me to focus on my own behavior and the root causes of my cravings. One I knew the cause of my unhealthy cravings, I found ways not just to satiate those feelings—but to make myself feel genuinely stronger and healthier.

- **Love.** I didn't expect this as an outcome, but this program fosters love. Weird, huh? It made me more loving, and I felt more connected to the world and people around me.

- **Freedom.** The more I delved into ancient secrets, the old societal paradigm started to slip off my shoulders. I didn't feel constrained.

- **Relationships.** As a result of this program, an entirely new world has opened up to me. I have friends across the globe who are always willing to talk with me and help me discover new truths. The holistic health practitioner network has become an extended family, one that I love dearly.

- **Better sleep.** Immediately, I could sleep through the nights, which is something I've always struggled with before. I developed control of my mind, and in the process, I could flip the switch to stop my mind from racing so I could slumber.

- **Improved mood.** I wouldn't say that I was a card-carrying asshole before taking this program, but I'm happy to admit that my general mood has improved greatly. I'm more calm, less reactive. I'm able to approach situations with more detachment, instead of letting circumstances hijack my emotions.

It doesn't matter if you're a medical professional, intellectually curious, a professional hobbyist, or someone with the heart of a healer, this program gets you started.

A quick word to those wanting to add *Certified Holistic Health Practitioner* to your existing credentials and body of work. When I started to fuel my own operation, I remember the unknowns and uncertainty as to the best next step. Rest assured, I did the hard work of trial and error, so you don't have to. I've spent the time to make it easier for those getting started. I'll even help you with tips along the way that you might not expect from a holistic health practitioner program. (For example, I was once a financial advisor, so I know a bit about running a fiscally responsible business! And I'm currently CFO at ProPride Industries, in the transportation industry) I'll share insight whenever I can.

If we don't offer a service now, chances are, we will soon (maybe even by the time you read this). For example, as of press time for this book, I can help fuel your online sales, where you can add a shopping cart on your website for products, and I'll take care of the inventory, shipping, and stock. I've had this in the works for quite a while, and I'm nearly ready to launch.

And if you're a professional wanting consulting on your marketing, that's in the works, too. If you're looking for a turnkey operation, I will set you up with the right tools, structure, and know-how to make that happen. If you want to build your own, I'm right there if you need anything. You can do as much or as little on your own as you can handle. Either way, I can support you, and you'll never be alone.

CHAPTER 9

THE TURNKEY VERSUS THE DIY HOLISTIC HEALTH PRACTITIONER BUSINESS PRACTICE

"A strong spirit transcends rules."

Prince

If you're considering becoming a holistic health practitioner, you are probably planning how you will start and run your business. Let me ask you one of the most pressing questions: would you rather operate a turnkey operation—or build your own from the ground up?

Let me start with the DIY option. Some people think, *"Well, if I do it myself, I don't have to pay consultants. So it will be cheaper. And it'll be easier, since I won't have to listen to anyone telling me what I have to do."* Perhaps, but there's an old saying, "We all pay for our education. No matter where we get it, we always pay for it." I can tell you from building my own clinic that it isn't the same place today as the one I started out to build. I made mistakes. I spent a lot of money learning those lessons. Heck, I didn't know what I didn't know, and how I paid for that! Yup, I paid for my education.

If you put your heart and soul into making your DIY operation successful, and you're willing to lose some sleep in the process, you'll get it done eventually. But as I said, you'll pay for your education either now or later.

Recently, I read a book on the attributes of world-class leaders. Several of the leaders in that book mentioned how critical it is to find mentors, consultants, gurus, and mastermind groups to accelerate their learning. Here's a silly example to make the point. Let's say I had an old classic Mustang convertible with a carburetor instead of the modern fuel injection that's now the norm. If I wanted to rebuild the carburetor on that old Mustang, I'd go to YouTube, read books and manuals, and tap into my local auto parts store to figure out how to do it. But what's the point? I'd have less personal interest in learning how to rebuild a carburetor than I'd have in getting my old Mustang purring like a kitten while I'm driving it. So just because I *could do it* doesn't mean it would be the best investment of my limited time. Does that make sense?

Likewise, if you're committed to building your own business, you'll figure it out. But ask yourself if you're more interested in figuring out how to *develop* your own business—or are you more passionate about *optimally operating* your business?

If you choose to build your own business, you will need a plan. What makes that so challenging is that when you've never done it before, it's very challenging to set goals and develop a growth strategy. Maybe you say, "I want one hundred new customers each month by the end of year." Great! Now let me pose some questions for you to consider:

- *How will you get there?*
- *Do you have a population size that makes those numbers attainable?*
- *What's your marketing budget?*
- *How about your marketing strategies?*
- *If you were to reach that growth, do you have a staffing model to accommodate that demand?*
- *Do you have a website?*
- *Will you be taking appointments from your website?*

• Will you sell additional products and services on your website? In your office?

• Will you need to build a new, or retrofit an existing, building site?

Those are just some questions you must consider before developing your goals. I had to figure all of this out on my own.

Building a business is a full-time job, one that has almost nothing to do with the healing arts. Unless you have the stomach and heart for this kind of endeavor, consider the second option: a turnkey operation.

Next, let me say a bit about the turnkey and mentoring options, and why they are the way to go for many practitioners. I understand the ins and outs of setting up and operating, and I can advise you very well on how things should work.

With my *turnkey program*, I help build or reconstruct your website customized to you, your business, and your practice. Think of the website as a working template. I've worked with enough business consultants to know what belongs and what doesn't. So I offer a robust template that works extremely well. The beauty of the website is that you will have a portal to order from—or from which you can show your clients how to order for themselves. Right from the website, you can order items that will ship to your office or directly to your client.

In addition to the website, I include a weekly video call with either me or an expert on my end on any particular aspect of the business you want to learn about. Over time, those calls become bi-weekly, and then monthly. Obviously, we want to offer you as much support as possible on the front end, when every experience is new and more intense. Once you settle in, we make those video calls less frequent.

You can sign up for either 12, 24, or 36 months for the turnkey program. At times, we make the engagement shorter than 12 months, once you demonstrate that you've gotten the hang of things. We will teach you how to write proposals, create your own marketing copy, even show you how to design your own flyers. If you're interested, we'll teach how to complete all forms, waivers, procedures. You can even work on your own books. With our turnkey program, everything is planned. No surprises on your end. We will schedule with you to meet weekly, monthly, quarterly, or annually. Our aim is to make your success feel easy.

We also have a very strong *mentoring program,* which is more highly customized to your specific goals and needs. Remote mentoring can be challenging, but I've done it long enough to make it work well for our partners. With our monthly mentoring program, you'll meet with me or one of my designees. We encourage mentees to submit questions via email or even video that we will tackle on the video mentoring session. You might have a question about something tactical, like, "How do I complete this part of an intake form?" Or you might have a strategic question, like "If you're looking to expand, which regions offer the greatest need?" If you are near my office, you can even join me while I answer questions for others as a way to accelerate your learning even more.

One difference between turnkey and mentoring is that our turnkey sessions are planned, whereas our mentoring sessions are ad hoc and per your request.

This isn't my first rodeo, so to speak. I've been in the healing arts for long enough to have friends and associates across the world from some of the oldest institutions for holistic healing out there. And I can tell you without fear of contradiction that no other institute in the United States that I know of offers as many options for their students and graduates as we do. I'm very proud of that. While it took me years to get where I am today, this Institute feeds two of my greatest joys: one, promoting natural, holistic healing; and two, helping like-minded holistic healing professionals succeed.

CHAPTER 10

LEAD THE CHANGE BY TAKING CHARGE

"We are continually telling ourselves and the Universe that we are healthy, or we are not."

David D. Jameson, DNM

Doctor of Natural Medicine

The Blue Lotus Institute for Holistic Studies is a godsend for those who want personal growth. I read a statistic the other day that said 98 percent of changes that we try to institute in our lives fail to stick. Read that again. Ninety-eight percent of them fail. And the reason they fail is because our programming—the narrative that we've heard and accepted about ourselves for years—keeps us stuck. So no matter how badly we desire change, we have years and years of programming that snap us right back where we started.

I'll be vulnerable and share an example from my own weakness. A while back, I told myself that I would start each morning with a thirty-minute walk. And it worked great. For a time. Then one morning, I talked myself out of it. Old programming took over. So I skipped my walk. But the next morning, I jumped right back on the horse, and I walked again. However, the morning after that, I told myself, "Look, maybe doing it every day is a bit too much. I think it should be every other day instead." So I skipped that day. Act surprised when I tell you that within a week, I stopped walking.

That is how programming works. To fight that programming, we have to recondition and reprogram our neural pathways that are ingrained in our psyches.

That's why it's so hard to break bad eating habits. Ironically, eating the things that we're addicted to makes it harder to stop eating the things that we're addicted to. It's a vicious cycle, one that makes us drawn to the things that make us sick as human beings. So just like with my failed walking habit, I made up a story in my head as to why it was okay to change the plan. So I changed it, and nothing bad happened. Except I became one of the 98 percent of changes that don't stick. Once I broke the programming and reprogrammed my thinking about my morning walks, I not only go on those walks now, but I thoroughly enjoy them!

When you are ready to *be the change*, as Ghandi implored, you'll understand how your mind works at a whole new level. For example, you'll be able to sense six distinct tastes: sweet, sour, salty, bitter, pungent, and astringent. Most people have an addiction to sweet and salty. Here's where our minds and old programming keep us stuck. Think back to when you were a child. Did your mom ever celebrate your greatest accomplishments with special foods? That's what many parents do. They show love and reward their children with yummy foods. The most common food "rewards" seem to be pizza and ice cream. Once we start to associate appreciation and love with food, our programming becomes entrenched. Over time, whenever you achieve something special, you tell yourself, *"Do you know what? I deserve pizza and ice cream! I've earned it!"* And now, years later, you've established a pattern—one that equates success with foods linked in inflammation and obesity. Is it any wonder that people struggle to make changes in their lives, when so much of their programming lies buried so deeply in the psyches?

That's why outside-in changes fail. That's why we say, "I'm going to start a diet. I'll start next Monday!" And that's why we fail. Unless we go deep inside to uncouple our programming, our entrenched bad habits will always win. Human beings choose a familiar misery (like feeling bloated, sluggish, and overweight) over unfamiliar happiness, because our neural pathways run like endless miles of train tracks in our heads. Most of the time, we wake up in the morning, and we are already on the train rails. It's familiar. We don't question it. It's completely normal to us.

Even when we know that we have become slaves to miserable, unhealthy habits, those habits form the path of least resistance. To get off the track means to find a way to break the track. The crux of all holistic medicine is being able to do something different. If nothing changes, nothing changes.

I often use food addiction as an example, because nearly everyone relates to it. But did you know our minds and bodies can become addicted to just about anything? Some people are addicted to watching or reading the news. It doesn't matter if the news is good (it seldom is), bad, fake, local, or whatever. People don't realize that a "news addiction" is nothing more than an anger addiction—which is simply a hormone addiction. When you read something that gets your blood boiling, cortisol floods your body, similar to the endorphin high that runners experience. We crave hormone release.

Unhealthy addictions, ones that usually stem from early experiences, prevent people from making positive changes in their lives. Holistic health practitioners learn how to reprogram their own minds first. Once practitioners experience the freedom of living life addiction free, they become natural evangelists for the holistic crusade.

World-class holistic health practitioners perceive the things around them differently than most people. Armed with a healthy perspective, they flood themselves with positive mantras and self-talk. Positive self-talk equips the best healers to defeat their broken, self-defeating thoughts—the same programming that blocks change. Finally, once they've added to the arsenal the best learning (starting with Ayurvedic teachings), they have the skills to practice better routines. All of these skills operating together form a most powerful healing system that encompasses the practitioner's life and work.

A friend called me the other day to admit he'd slipped into some unhealthy habits. He told me, "David, I just need more willpower." Hogwash! Professor of psychology at the University of Toronto and the principal investigator at the Toronto Laboratory for Social Neuroscience, Michael Inzlicht, found that willpower—just like anger, joy, and other emotions—ebbs and flows throughout the day based on what's happening around us. Do you see why willpower alone isn't enough to drive behavioral change? Lasting change starts with replacing old thoughts with new ones, old foods with new ones, old activities with new ones. And it all starts with thoughts, not emotions. I don't always *feel* like making wise, healthy food choices. But I don't have to give into my emotions. I've retrained my brain and thinking so eating healthy, natural foods (which I know is the right thing to do) actually releases hormones in my body that create positive emotions.

If you would lead the change in the lives of others, you must take charge of your own mind first.

I remember being down in the Florida Keys and visiting an herbalist. I'm not making this up; he was the biggest man I've ever seen in real life. He stood about 6 feet 10 inches and easily weighed 400 pounds. I'm dead serious when I say that he had to stoop and turn sideways to get through the front door. Oh, and did I mention he arrived 15 minutes late to our appointment? I went to see him, because I wanted to ask him a few questions and purchase a few things at his shop. But I ended up walking out without saying a word or purchasing a thing.

Why would I take advice and patronize a business run by someone with such little self-control? How can he offer a better way to live to those wanting to make positive change, when he's not even able to *be the change* for himself? Successful holistic health practitioners walk the walk and talk the talk. They've worked on themselves, and it shows in the way they carry themselves, care for themselves, and demonstrate care for others.

Are you ready to *be the change*? Are you ready to *lead the change*? Are you ready to *take charge of your life* in every way imaginable? Are you ready to become a *real holistic health practitioner?* If you answered yes to any of these questions—or even a strong maybe—it's time to learn how to do it (and finally hear about that free offer I mentioned in the Introduction).

CONCLUSION
HERE'S MY FREE GIFT TO YOU—$250 VALUE

This is the part of the book that stops being about me, and starts being about you. I've shared with you a bit of my journey—and what we infuse in everyone at the Blue Lotus Institute for Holistic Studies.

But remember, *when nothing changes, nothing changes*. And the best person to willingly change your life is YOU.

- *Are you tired of living half a life, running on empty, chasing the pill or next cure?*
- *Do you wish you could offer your patients, clients, or family members*

something more to enhance their healing—and elevate their lives?

- *Are you craving to learn the age-old mysteries to unlock greater wellness?*
- *Do you want your own life to be filled with more vibrancy, connection, love, energy, and fulfillment?*
- *Do you long to leave a health legacy that your kids will respect—and emulate?*

If you answered yes to any of these questions, I invite you to take the next step, which is to ACCEPT MY GIFT. Since you've invested your time in reading this book, I'm willing to give something back—which is *my own time.*

For the limited run-time of this book edition, I offer you a FREE, no-obligations, 15-minute call with yours truly. This comes at a $250 value to you, absolutely free. You can use our time to discuss a health issue, if you want. But my hope is that you will ask me about our Certified Holistic Health Practitioner program at Blue Lotus Institute for Holistic Studies. I'm an open book to share any and all information to help you become a healer—which will save you money in the long run.

If you think you don't yet know enough to invest in yourself, or aren't qualified, think again. There are NO prerequisites to get on the phone with me—or enroll in our program. In fact, I'd love it if everyone would enroll! Anyone with a passion for wellness deserves to live fully, and the best way to do that is to learn the ancient—and modern—secrets to holistic health.

<u>Regardless if you wish to add **Certified Holistic Health Practitioner** to your current chiropractic practice, massage therapy practice, health food store business, or if you're simply trying to find natural, effective ways to care for</u>

your family, what you will learn at the Institute will transform your life—and the lives around you—forever.

NEXT STEP: Call me at 800-385-8371, or visit www.bluelotushealingcenter.com to schedule a FREE call with me, or learn more about our Certified Holistic Health Practitioner program.

If you choose to enroll, remember, you can take the classes from anywhere, on the convenience of your computer. Even the timeframe is flexible, accommodating those who work full-time or have other commitments. You will walk away with a certificate of accreditation you can hang on the wall to show your clients, customers, and friends. But more than that, *you will hold the power to heal yourself of the stresses and illnesses that have held you back from your best.*

You don't have to enroll, but I still owe you a FREE gift. Contact me today, and I promise to make our discussion worthwhile.

Sincerely in health,

David D. Jameson, DNM
Doctor of Natural Medicine
Certified Ayurvedic Practitioner
Certified Holistic Health Practitioner
Clinic: www.bluelotushealingcenter.com
810.620.1000
Blue Lotus Institute for Holistic Studies
www.holistichealthpractitioner.com
800.385.8371

ABOUT THE AUTHOR

David has roots as a holistically minded young man dating back decades. David's mother tells stories of how when he was a young boy, he would talk about being an American Indian medicine man and having visions of using plants and other natural items to heal people. Throughout David's life, he has always been "that guy" you could call and ask a healing type question, as he has been well read in ancient healing teachings and homeopathy for almost four decades. As he was self-taught in homeopathy, David has treated himself, friends and family naturally for a long time just to be helpful, caring and to spread the love found in holistic healing. David decided to make holistic medicine his profession and started on a quest of study that has taken him to many states, and even India. This journey has required a vast commitment not only in time and finances for study programs, doctoral studies, internships, and trips abroad, but a sacrifice to the profession he loves. David was awarded the doctoral degree of DNM, Doctor of Natural Medicine. David's true love is Ayurveda, and he's also worked in India under a famous Ayurvedic doctor in the traditional setting of guru-to-student, and not university teachings. Ayurveda is a life-long journey and requires a discipline that continues to evolve due to its vastness. Now as an Ayurvedic Practitioner and Doctor of Natural Medicine, David is seeing people at his clinic, Blue Lotus Healing Center (BLHC), and also teaches Holistic Health Practitioners and beginning Ayurvedic Consultants though his institute, Blue Lotus Institute for Holistic Studies, located in the same center as BLHC.

David D. Jameson, DNM
Doctor of Natural Medicine
Certified Ayurvedic Practitioner
Certified Holistic Health Practitioner
Clinic: www.bluelotushealingcenter.com
810.620.1000
Blue Lotus Institute for Holistic Studies
www.holistichealthpractitioner.com
800.385.8371

www.ingramcontent.com/pod-product-compliance
Lightning Source LLC
Chambersburg PA
CBHW071557270726
48657CB00026B/571